The
BORAX
BOOK

Incredible Uses for Borax

N.D. Lorenz

Welcome to the Borax Book. From the writer of <u>Borax Girl</u> comes the research of the incredible uses of the product Borax - a quick guide to this amazing product. Banned by pharmaceutical giants in other countries when they discovered how great it really is and could not be patented, we are grateful to still have this "laundry booster" available to us, and at such a reasonable price, on our store shelves in America.

Contents

Borax for Health

Starting with the important stuff.

* An analysis from the Chemical Regulatory Consulting Board states that, "Boric acid [Borax] is only poisonous if taken internally or inhaled in large quantities." You would need to consume around a full cup of Borax for toxicity, and 1/8 tsp is generally enough per day for the entirety of the ailment.

Arthritis. Any joint pain and inflammation can be lessoned and/or cured by simply adding a pinch of Borax to a warm or hot drink any time of the day, once per day.

Bone strengthening. Because we are lacking in all minerals, and boron works in conjunction with calcium, a pinch of Borax will gradually strengthen your bones.

Brittle Bone Disease. See above.

Osteoporosis. See above.

Joints. This speaks to inflammation, and will be noticed slowly over time.

Balances hormones. Boron, and Borax is an easy way to get it, is a necessary element in our bodies. We have over 20 different hormones in our very complex bodies, and a pinch of Borax per day helps to balance them.

Menstrual cramping. See above.

Neutron absorber. Borax helps remove toxins and balance a myriad of problems.

Anti-fungal medication. Kills candida fungus – used on nail fungus, and can kill more drug-resistant forms of candida glabrada.

Cancer treatment (as one tool of many, not alone!), specifically melanoma, breast cancer, and prostate cancer – hormone-driven cancers.

Ear drops. Effective antibiotic for the treatment of ear infections and pain relief.

Eye drops. Common ingredient in eye drops, but safe in very small doses as a home remedy in distilled water.

Yeast infections.

Vaginitis [infection].

Fungal ailments of the skin and organs.

Memory loss. This may be from the removal of infections in the body, allowing the brain to function better and/or as it should.

Retention of Vitamin D, and therefore brain function.

Estrogen booster, hormone balancer.

Weight control. As a bonus side effect of all the uses listed above, when our hormones are balanced, our bodies function the way they are intended to and will return to their healthy state, including healthy "normal" weight.

Borax is good for you!

(In small doses, of course.)

Borax as a Cleaning Agent

Brightening of cotton – both in your washing machine and by hand for delicate cotton garments, of course.

Mold and fungus killer.

> Mix Borax with soap and water to make a fabulous cleaning solution.

Cutting boards, specifically wood cutting boards.

Scouring powder. Especially on copper-bottom pans and rust, but also for showers, tubs, and tiles.

Garbage disposal drain sanitizer.

Unclogging drains. Simply mix into boiling water and allow to sit and dissolve clog.

Carpet cleaner. Sprinkle into carpets, with or without baking soda, allow to sit, and then vacuum up.

Borax is a pest deterrent, but will not kill them.

Refreshening linens and mattresses.

Deodorizer. A pinch goes a long way to removing the smell from your garbage cans.

Stainless steel stains, and porcelain stains. A paste of Borax with lemon juice work wonders.

More Uses for Borax

Fertilizer – boric acid is a crucial nutrient for all plant life, too.

Feed fruit trees, including tomatoes.

Finishing of cotton in textile factories.

Forging metal.

Soldering metal welding.

Flame and fire retardants.

Cleaners, of course. □

Slime for playing. The easy recipe is:

    1 Tbsp Borax

    1 cup water (distilled)

    White glue, 8 oz. bottle (Elmer's)

    Food coloring

Prevents wilting of flowers while drying for preservation.

Fun Facts

Anyone wear contacts or use eye drops? Borax is an ingredient in both.

Just a reminder – a pinch (1/8 tsp) has no flavor and dissolves instantly.

Boron is the 5th Element on the Periodic Table.

Boron [Boric acid and Borax] is mined in Death Valley and today there is a Visitor's Center and museum in the town of Boron, CA.

Borax is non-toxic in small doses.

Not so fun fact: Borax will not kill ticks, bed bugs, lice, spiders, beetles, flies, fleas, or moths. Sorry.

If a fish tank is dirty,
clean the tank, don't
drug the fish.

Blessings!

www.ingramcontent.com/pod-product-compliance
Lightning Source LLC
Chambersburg PA
CBHW071555260726
48653CB00008BA/3278